The
Roller Coaster Ride
of
Alzheimer's/
Dementia

The Roller Coaster Ride of Alzheimer's/ Dementia

Pavah Kucharek

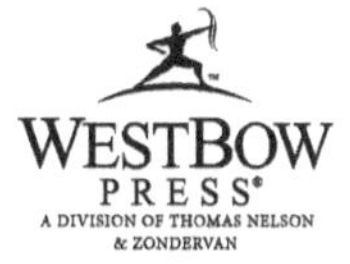

WESTBOW
PRESS®
A DIVISION OF THOMAS NELSON
& ZONDERVAN

WestBow Press books may be ordered through booksellers or by contacting:

WestBow Press
A Division of Thomas Nelson & Zondervan
1663 Liberty Drive
Bloomington, IN 47403
www.westbowpress.com
1 (866) 928-1240

Because of the dynamic nature of the Internet, any web addresses or
links contained in this book may have changed since publication and
may no longer be valid. The views expressed in this work are solely those
of the author and do not necessarily reflect the views of the publisher,
and the publisher hereby disclaims any responsibility for them.

Any people depicted in stock imagery provided by Getty Images are models,
and such images are being used for illustrative purposes only.
Certain stock imagery © Getty Images.

ISBN: 978-1-9736-4308-1 (sc)
ISBN: 978-1-9736-4309-8 (e)

Library of Congress Control Number: 2018912427

Print information available on the last page.

WestBow Press rev. date: 10/26/2018

For Mom

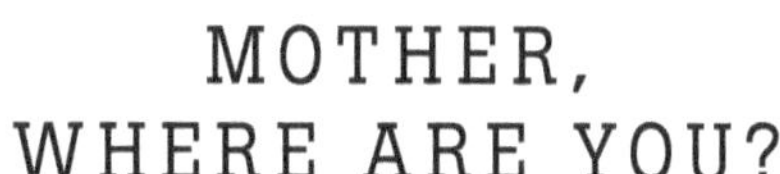

MOTHER, WHERE ARE YOU?

Mother, where are you?
Where did you go?
You left me so slowly,
But still here to show.

Mother, where are you?
I look for you everywhere.
I yearn for your eyes to look at me
Instead of a dead-straight stare.

Mother, where are you?
As I hold you, I want a hug
But know you stiffen from fear
Of this stranger's touch or tug.

Mother, where are you?
Do you dream of days gone by?
Am I your child again in dreams?
Or has this evil robbed them dry?

Mother, where are you?
I miss you so!
To have you right in front of my eyes,
But then, not to have you at all …

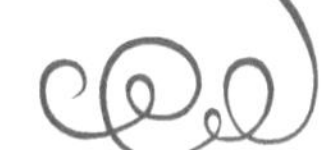

CHAPTER 1

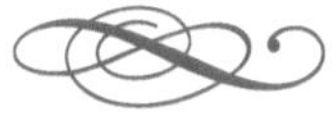

When walking up to a roller coaster ride for the first time, how do you know how much fun or how scary it will be? Everyone reacts differently, I suppose, waiting in line with anticipation and butterflies in their stomachs. What lies ahead? You can see it has some ups and downs and turns, but how are you going to be able to take them? I'm a little afraid but excited too! I think some will laugh, some will scream, and some will even cry.

On my personal roller coaster ride, I have done all the above and more. I have found this to be the only way to truly describe the journey I have been on with my mother, who has had dementia for over eighteen years. She is ninety-seven and in the final stage of this disease of the mind. The beginning of the disease is like standing in line, waiting to get in the car on this roller coaster ride. What lies ahead of you and your loved one is a mystery, and the unknown ride ahead is a bit daunting. You can read all the books on the disease you can, and I have read ten or twelve, but I have found over the years there are no cookie-cutter symptoms, actions, or upcoming behaviors you can totally rely on. In other words, some people with dementia may act totally different than others.

Since my sister and I lived over an hour away from our parents and still worked, and my brother was retired but lived almost three hours away, my sister and I went to see them on the weekends or had them over to our houses for visits. Both my parents were still driving. My father was eighty-one when he started complaining about my mother forgetting things and putting items away and not being able to find them again. She was probably around seventy-five at the time. Not having any real experience with dementia (other than my grandma being "senile," and reportedly having hardening of the carotid artery), we just thought it was part of the aging process. So we took my mother to the doctor, and she passed the short dementia test. We just let it go as just normal aging. We noticed little things, but being unfamiliar with the disease, we ignored the symptoms and thought my dad was also exaggerating a little. Mother complained about my dad being forgetful too!

CHAPTER 2

The first part of the roller coaster's big drop came when my father died two years later. My mother had lived alone in her house for about six months, and we went to see her every weekend to visit with her, put her medication in her pill boxes, and pay her bills. My dad had always done everything for her, and she didn't know how to even pay a bill.

We knew the time was coming when we would have to move her out of her house and take her car away. But we didn't realize how soon it would be. She had friends over every week to have lunch and play cards. After they left one time, Mother decided to go to the grocery store. Two of the women were standing by one of their cars parked in the driveway, talking. Mother didn't open the garage door until she got into her car and opened it with the garage door clicker on her visor. Without looking in her rearview mirror, she started her car, and despite the women yelling, she didn't hear them and gunned the car in reverse, smashing into the woman's car parked behind her.

As I said before, my sister and I still worked full time, and only seeing her on the weekends did not give us a true picture of how she was mentally declining. We talked to her on the phone every day, but that gave no indication of how she was doing mentally. She could fake a conversation very well!

So now came the time to take her car away and move her out of her home to a senior center apartment complex. That was a big fight, but we won this time due to the accident, and she was becoming afraid of living by herself. And some of her friends already lived in the complex she was moving to.

But after the move, over the next year, she started having panic attacks and calling my sister in the middle of the night, saying she was having a heart attack and had already called 911 to pick her up. She'd had two heart attacks years earlier and was afraid she was having another one. Her second heart attack had ended up with open-heart surgery and a double bypass. My sister would call me and say Mother had called again with fears of having another episode. So we would travel an hour from each area we lived to the ER for all the tests and an overnight stay for the same results. The panic attacks started happening more frequently, until she was calling every other week over a period of four months. It became exhausting when you had to work the next day.

The icing on the cake and the decision to move her in with the three of us on a rotating basis was when she started overtaking her medication. One day she left the stove on and started a fire. I'm sure the owners of the senior apartment complex were also happy with our decision. Her friends told us she was forgetting where her room was and would forget their names, and they had to help her play cards.

We took her to the doctor, a geriatric physician, to be tested again for dementia, and this time she failed miserably. This time she didn't even remember the doctor's name. My mother was diagnosed with dementia. At the time of her diagnosis, the only way a person could be definitely diagnosed with Alzheimer's was after death via autopsy of the brain. Although you kind of know your loved one has the disease, when you hear it from the doctor, it still makes your knees buckle. You know, but you don't want to hear it.

CHAPTER 3

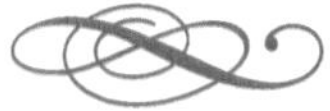

After this hard fall on the roller coaster, it goes very slowly up the next hill. This was the way it was with my mother in the beginning. She functioned fairly well, and it was a slow roller coaster ride for about eight years. We began by moving all her belongings between my two siblings' houses and my house, and taking turns having her live with each of us for a couple of months at a time. I retired early, my brother was retired, and my sister still worked but had help when my mother was at her house. My sister took care of all her medical needs, and I took care of her bills and everything else. Mother seemed happy, and it worked out fairly well for us, except when she tried to go for a walk outside in the middle of the night, and the alarm started screeching at 2:00 a.m. So you learn to become very inventive on where to put an extra lock that your loved one cannot reach.

My mother has always been a very good Christian who loved her family, her church, and everyone around her. She would always see some good in anyone she met. We have been blessed that she has kept her sweetness during this disease. At one point, she didn't want to eat very much and just wanted to sleep all the time. She talked in her sleep, so when she was at my brother's house, he decided to record her conversations. Most of it was gibberish, but one time she was having a serious conversation with my teenage daughter, whom she called by name. Mother was sitting on the side of the bed with her eyes closed and her arm out, as if she were holding on to my daughter next to her. She was telling her to always be a good girl when it came to boys. Mother said, "Now listen to me, sweetie, I know that you are pretty, and you dress very nice. But boys are after just one thing, and I don't want you to forget that. Are you listening to your grandma? Okay, always remember that pretty is as pretty does." This went on for about an hour and a half as she preached to my now forty-year-old daughter. My brother has several tapes that are precious to us of her talking about different things to who knows who she is speaking to. But this one was so special because she called out my daughter's name. It is so wonderful to have her voice on tape forever.

It took some time to get her appetite back and get her up and out of bed from sleeping so much. But her confusion continued to grow. She started finding it harder and harder to find the right words to use. It was a fight to give her a shower, and she wasn't happy with any of us. She was not steady on her feet, and we had to get her a walker. This went on until none of us could physically take care of her needs anymore.

My sister and I started shopping for assisted living/memory care facilities. We decided on a place close to my sister since she was a nurse and could get to Mother quickly if anything medically happened. We found a place just fifteen minutes away from my sister. The only problem with that was I was still an hour away, and my brother was still three hours away. But we felt it was more important that my mother be closer to my sister.

CHAPTER 4

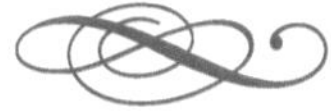

Hold on to your hats, the roller coaster has come to the top of another hill and is getting ready to fall! Now comes the time to tell your loved one who has dementia that he or she has the disease and is going to an assisted living facility. Not fun, not pretty, and then you get the proverbial, "Nothing is wrong with me, and why are you doing this to your mother?" Funny, she seems to have her mind together at the most inopportune moment! We took this fall on the roller coaster hard and yelled all the way down! Ladies and gentlemen, if ever my mother had a clearer mind, it was this entire day. She preached the entire time as we were driving that nothing was wrong with her, she didn't need to go to *that* place, and so on. I tried to explain to her why she did and how much better it would be for her. Once she got there, walked in with her little walker, saw other residents with walkers and wheelchairs, saw her apartment with her furniture and clothes, and met the people, she settled down. It only took her a couple of weeks to start bossing everyone around like she did us. It became her new home.

Over the next two years, this was the part of the roller coaster that took the small dips up and down and around curves. She would forget where her room was even though her name was on the door, and she had no concept of time. She needed assistance with every part of her daily living. I still took care of her bills, took her to the doctor, eye doctor, out to eat, and so on. My sister took care of her medication ordering and seeing her when she was able, and my brother came and took her out to eat and brought her candy when he could. She enjoyed playing bingo but always needed help because of her failing eyesight and hearing. So I tried to go three times a week to help her play her favorite game and eat lunch with her. Alzheimer's and dementia rob individuals not only of their brains but of their eyesight, hearing, and so much more.

As a caregiver, and on the roller coaster ride of dementia, you must have that humor button you can push at all times. Pretty funny things sometimes come out in conversations. My mother, who never smoked in her life, for some reason started asking me for a cigarette when we went out to the patio or took a walk. I asked her why, after all these years of yelling at everyone else about smoking, she would start now. She replied, "Because I can!" I figured at ninety years old, what was it going to hurt now? And the funny thing about this was, her mother, my grandma, had dementia (back then we called it "senility") and did the exact same thing. Grandma also hated smoking, but she smoked a little longer than my mother. My mother smoked about two months. My grandma smoked over a year because everyone else was doing it, so she wanted to smoke too.

Mother loved to gossip about the residents and how gaudily they decorated their walkers and wheelchairs. Her walker was decorated, but you couldn't see it. When you lifted up the seat of her walker, it was full of plates, melted chocolate, cookies, cake—whatever she had eaten for lunch or dinner the day before—bead necklaces, stuffed animals … you get the idea. It was overflowing every time I went there. She fussed at me the whole time I was cleaning it out and washing the chocolate off the bottom because she was afraid I would throw something good away. I even found other women's jewelry and men's underwear—yes, men's underwear! I asked her who she visited at night, and she wouldn't tell me. You have got to laugh, people! I always laughed when I left the room to get something. And when I came back in, my mother greeted me like I just arrived, no matter how many times I did it. Again, you have to laugh; otherwise you're going to cry an awful lot. Always keep your humor.

CHAPTER 5

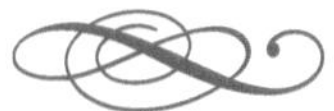

Out of the blue, a big loop-de-loop came on the roller coaster. I came out of my seat, but the bar held me in. I got another middle-of-the-night phone call, around 3:30 a.m., but it wasn't about my mother this time. It was my brother-in-law, telling me my sister was in a coma and that I had to come quick to the hospital ER. What? I had just talked to her that afternoon, and I knew she was having trouble with her blood pressure. I had begged her to let me take her to the ER, but she refused because she was going to the doctor the next day. She had so much fluid in her lungs she was gurgling, but being a nurse, she knew when the time would come for her to go to the hospital. She said she would go when her husband got home, if necessary. I begged her to no avail. I've never forgiven myself for not just going over to her house, making her get in the car, and taking her to the doctor or the ER. The last thing I did for her was make her laugh out loud. But that wasn't what I wanted to do!

I got to the hospital ER, and they decided to airlift her to a better hospital and put her in intensive care. She never woke from her coma, and the tests they performed a few days later showed no brain activity. So we made the hard decision as a family to stop all life support two days before my mother's birthday. We had already planned a big party the following weekend, and I didn't want my sister to die on my mother's actual birth date. But my sister lived those two days and died on my mother's birthday. I've never been able to celebrate my mother's birthday on her real birth date since. She was not just my sister but my right arm and best friend. It's been eight years, and I'm still not over her sudden, unexpected death. Never will be. But I look forward to the day I see her again in heaven.

Due to my mother's dementia, we did not tell her about my sister being in the hospital, and she had not asked why she had not seen her. To my mother, my sister had pretty much become out of sight, out of mind at this point. We asked her doctor how we should tell her about my sister's death. Being a geriatric physician and having more experience with things like this, we felt he knew her well enough to give us the best advice. He suggested it was entirely up to us, but in his opinion, we should not tell her because it could go really badly, and she might totally fixate on it the rest of her life. As a family, we talked it over and had a difference of opinion. But we went with the doctor's advice and decided not to tell her. It turned out to be the right decision.

One time after my sister passed, I had all the family over for a holiday meal and Mother said, "It seems like someone's missing." We just talked around it and changed the subject. We told the staff at her assisted living facility that we did not tell her about my sister's death, and if she ever asked for my sister, they were to call me. This happened one evening about four months later. I got a call around ten o'clock, and they told me Mother was asking for my sister. My mother got on the phone with me and said she had just got off the train and was in a place she did not know, and to come get her and take her home. I tried my best to explain to her that she must have had a dream, and that was where she lived now. I felt so bad for her; the panic in her voice was gut-wrenching. She really was scared, and this was the first time I ever heard my mother deep-down scared. I just wanted to hold her and make it better. I talked to her for a while and eased her down some. I told her I would come see her in the morning. I went to see her the next day, and she didn't remember any of it.

I have become the major caregiver for my mother since she went into assisted living, and as you will learn later, due to circumstances beyond all our control, her only caregiver.

CHAPTER 6

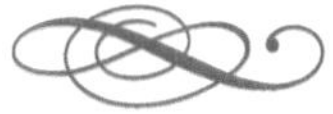

This upcoming part of the roller coaster came as a large hill after a huge curve. Mother's memory kept declining over the next six months, and I knew the time would be coming soon for her to need memory care. I received a call six months later from the assisted living staff. Mother had walked away from the facility, and they were searching for her as we spoke. Needless to say, I jumped in my car and broke the speed limit all the way there. On my arrival, they had just found her. She had gone several blocks away to an apartment building and was knocking on doors until someone answered, and then asking if they would take her to Illinois. The resident of the apartment knew of the assisted living facility nearby and called them, and they came and picked her up. Mother was all red, sweating, out of breath, and scared. This happened to be August, so it was very hot. They were giving her lots of water to cool her off and taking her vital signs. The decision was made right then that she would be moved to memory care within the hour. We could not afford another incident of her walking away from the facility.

I tried to explain to her that she was going from her apartment to a new bedroom in a different building. When we took the tour, she was okay but noticed the difference in the residents immediately. She was sad, but I told her she would make new friends. It didn't help that she soon discovered everything was locked down there, though there was open access to the patio with a rock wall all around.

Mother stayed in this memory care for five years. Along the way, she declined, forgetting names and faces, including mine. But she still remembered the old times of her youth. She tried to hide her memory loss without success. When we asked her if she knew who a family member we brought to see her was, she would say, "Of course." Then when we asked her the person's name, she would say, "They know their own name!"

She was very cagy that way. You have to laugh at how smart our loved ones are sometimes in covering up their forgetfulness, and the excuses they make.

Her health and mind both went down that long drop on the roller coaster. Her legs could no longer hold her weight, even though both were getting lighter at the same time, so she had to go into a wheelchair. I continued to get late-night calls when she tried to get out the locked doors and fell out of her wheelchair and got hurt. Again I rushed to her side in the middle of the night.

Another big snake in the roller coaster and then a drop came one day at 6:15 a.m. I received a call from the morning nurse that Mother had a bump on her head and was already on her way to the ER. *Wait a minute—how did this happen? A bump on the head, and she is on the way to the ER?* I thought. To the best of their knowledge, it seemed she must have fallen out of bed and now had a goose egg on her forehead. *Now it's a goose egg?* Then the nurse said, "We just want your mother checked over to make sure she is okay since she appears to have fallen somehow. It's just protocol." *You think?* Since I was an hour away and it was the beginning of morning traffic time, I just put on clothes—no makeup, no shower—and took off. I didn't even wait for a cup of coffee!

Ladies and gentlemen, when I arrived at the ER and saw how bad my mother looked and how swollen and cut up she was, I dropped to the floor. Bump on the head my butt! Her entire face was swollen, like she had fallen straight on her face. I had two nurses in the ER tell me that when she arrived, she was covered in dry blood, urine-soaked from head to toe, and the amount of swelling she had took several hours to occur. I was mad and horrified, crying for my mother because she didn't know what was going on and couldn't see anything because her eyes were swollen shut. Needless to say, an investigation was done. No one had checked on her since midnight the night before, so she must have lain there for about six hours. My mother had been in adult diapers for years. So for her to be urine-soaked from head to toe, I knew she had not been changed or checked on for hours.

After we got her back to her room from the hospital

and she took a shower, I went straight to the management, but the owners had conveniently left for the rest of the day. I requested their presence immediately, or I would call the authorities. Somehow, they were able to show up in ten minutes. To make a long story short, I got my point across and moved my mother closer to me, which is what I had planned to do anyway but not at her expense. I never blamed them for her fall, but they were supposed to check every resident every two hours, and according to the medical personnel, her swelling indicated it was much longer than two hours. And somehow the video for her hallway disappeared when requested by the governing bodies that be.

We moved my mother a month later. We found a very nice memory care place that only takes me fifteen minutes to get to, and they take such good care of my mother. They don't close the bedroom doors like the other place did, they have a beautiful patio for residents to use, and the nurses and common area are in the center where they can hear and see everything. I really like it, and somewhere deep inside, I know my mother does too.

CHAPTER 7

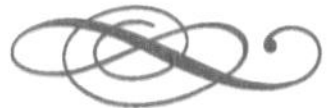

After the snake part of the ride came and went, a few dips and one big curve came around before we started going toward the end of the roller coaster. Mother seemed to settle in to her new surroundings fairly well. Her mind had deteriorated dramatically. I don't know if it was due to the fall, the move, or both. Over the next three months, she lost forty-five pounds and was put on hospice. We tried everything to get her to eat, but the only thing she really enjoyed were chocolate shakes. So that is what she got anytime she wanted them. Then, after about six months or so, ever so slowly, her mind continued to decline, but she decided she was hungry again and started to eat. A year after being on hospice and losing sixty pounds, she started eating like a little pig and gaining weight, and she came off hospice. Why a person has the will to live and turn around like that will always amaze me. Only the Lord knows the reason.

She comes out with some of the wildest things at times. She hallucinates more and more each day now. Mother tells me she sees little orange boys running around and playing by her. She sees my sister sometimes and my dad and my grandma. She sees little girls playing by her. She talks to them and asks them to come over and sit on her lap. She sundowns at times. That's when they get agitated in the evening and a little out of control. I've had calls in the evening from the staff when she has wanted to talk to her daughter. Once, she wanted me to come as soon as possible because the place was filling up with people, and there wouldn't be any seats left if I didn't get there right away. So I did the only thing I knew to do and told her I'd be there. I just didn't tell her a time.

She will talk and talk about nothing but get very agitated if you don't understand, so the best thing to do is always agree or disagree, depending on the conversation. Sometimes she gets in her "pass it on" mode, where every time she takes a bite of food, she wants to pass her plate to the next person. It is really hard to make her understand that she cannot share food with everyone at the table. Mother's mind functions as a child's now, and she doesn't understand that passing food on means passing germs on.

One of the aides was standing by her when I came in one day and said, "Oh, look, your daughter is here."

I bent down, looked her in the eyes, and said, "Hi, Mom."

She said, "That's no daughter of mine. She's too old!" Even though her eyesight is poor, in her mind I guess she is still young, and I should be too. Ouch, that hurt. I had to remind myself to laugh this time!

I went in one day and she was picking things out of the air. I asked what she was doing, and she replied, "Can't you tell?"

I guessed she was catching fireflies, but I was wrong. She was picking blackberries because she was making a blackberry pie. She asked, "Can't you see the crust over there?"

"Oh, yeah. I missed that when I came in I guess," I

muttered to myself. Another day I asked what she was doing, and she was churning butter. You never know where their minds wander.

When Mother is eating, she doesn't know how to use utensils anymore, or she doesn't know what to do next. She sits in front of her plate and asks me, "What should I do now?" I tell her to take a drink or take a bite. She has to eat finger foods because she can no longer see that well. When I am there at lunch or dinner, I feed her or put food on her fork or spoon for her to feed herself. She has trouble at the table and tries to eat her napkin and to eat food off of just a placemat. Sadly, her brain has become full of holes that no longer connect the dots due to this horrible disease. I try to help her every way I can.

Mother asked me one day out of the blue if she had any brothers and sisters. She is the oldest of seven, four girls and three boys. Two of her sisters are still living and have no signs of dementia. One brother passed from complications of dementia, and her mother had dementia. She used to remember her past but doesn't remember any of that anymore. She hasn't known me for nine years, doesn't remember my dad, and doesn't remember my siblings. She remembers nothing but what is happening in the moment, and then she is so confused about the moment. But every now and then, a spark will connect ever so quickly, and she remembers someone. Then it goes away in a microsecond. At times she stares off into space as if she is catatonic. Other times she talks nonstop and bosses everyone around.

I like to refer to my mother as my little box of chocolates. Whenever I go see her, I never know what I'm going to get! That's what life is all about anyway, right?

CHAPTER 8

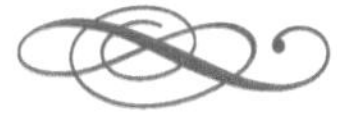

My brother had not been able to come see our mom for about four months. Back problems made him unable to make the three-hour drive. I understood because I had three back surgeries. He had all kinds of tests done, and they thought he had kidney stones, disk problems, and so on. Then he was not able to come see Mom for Christmas. A few days after Christmas, he called me and told me he was in the hospital. They had finally found out what was wrong with him; he had stage 4 pancreatic cancer. *Oh Lord, not again.* I thought. *Not my other sibling. My poor mother, who knows nothing that is going on, can hardly hear and can hardly see. This horrible disease has robbed her of her life. Please make me understand why this is happening again.* This was an unexpected upside-down turn on the roller coaster that I did not see coming!

They released him from the hospital. He decided not to take chemo because it would only buy him a couple more months of life, and he didn't want to go through all that for a few months. I made the drive to see him every week until he got delirium, and they put him in the hospice part of the hospital. Then I stayed with him the last ten days of his life. The time from diagnosis to death was only two and a half months. Very quick. I don't think any of us in the family were prepared, except for my brother. It gave us the opportunity to mend broken ties on my part from years ago, and I'm glad we had the brother-sister time together to do that. He was brave to the end. Now it is truly just my mother and me.

I had a huge pity party for myself after losing my brother. I kept it to myself the best I could, but I went into a depression and asked, "Why me? Why do I have all of this on my shoulders?"

The following month, I lost my best friend to cancer. The next month, my father-in-law was diagnosed with cancer. Now I'm his caregiver too. Then the next month I ended up in the hospital for six days with a bad case of diverticulitis. It was just beginning! My dog died suddenly the month after that, and we had a bad hurricane the following month. But when you least expect it, God speaks and you listen!

CHAPTER 9

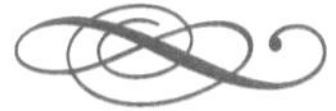

God brought me to my knees to have a talk one night and said, "Now do you see your pathway ahead? It's not about you; your mother is teaching you every day to have patience, compassion, love, and strength, and to share your experiences with others. You are becoming and will remain strong. Until now you've been the weakest one of the flock, but I will guide you from here on." And that is what I am doing. I am sharing my experiences the best way I can because God told me to. I was asked before to lead an Alzheimer's support group but refused because I always felt overwhelmed. Now I have renewed strength, energy, and love to help anyone in any way I can. I finally agreed to help a large, centrally organized Alzheimer's group as one of the support leaders in the assisted living/memory care facility where my mother is staying in now, and I'm very proud of that. The best advice I would give anyone who has a loved one with Alzheimer's or dementia is to attend a caregiver support group. You have the opportunity to meet people going through the same journey at different stages of the disease. They have a wealth of knowledge and can be a great deal of help. Trained counselors lead the meetings and have training and materials available. I have attended meetings and seminars for years, and it has helped me tremendously to hear other stories from first-time attendees, people who are still attending even after losing their loved ones, and even individuals who have been diagnosed with Alzheimer's or dementia. It will help you also. I promise.

The reason I use Alzheimer's/dementia is because some say they are one in the same. They are not, but the two have some of the same symptoms. We do know there is no cure at this time, and the end is the same for whatever your loved one has. There are medications out there that can keep a person at a certain level for a while, but there have not been any new medications in several years. My mother tried the medications for a few years, but they did not work for her. It is really up to the family to do their research and make informed decisions on what they want to do.

Our roller coaster ride is not over yet. I can see the end of it, but who knows what turns, loop-de-loops, or dips the Lord has ahead for my mother and me. Like I mentioned in the beginning of this book, my mother is ninety-seven, and we are in year eighteen of dementia. Looking back, I saw small symptoms two years before that, so let's say it's actually twenty years.

My hope for you is that your roller coaster ride is as smooth as possible, and that you love your Alzheimer's/dementia loved one with all your heart every day the Lord allows him or her to stay on this earth.

May God bless you.

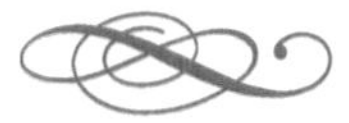

ABOUT THE AUTHOR

Pavah Kucharek enjoys living with her husband in their Central Florida home. She has three children and six grandchildren. She loves to travel and go on cruises with family and friends. She is also an avid reader. Pavah also volunteers at an Alzheimer's support group and is certified to lead group meetings. Her goal is to inform and help other families going through the emotional and mental struggle of this horrible disease.